Brews and Potions

Brews and Potions

A Hand Book of Remedies, Spells, Elixirs, Cordialls and Aphrodisiacs

Compiled and Introduced by

MAURICE RICKARDS

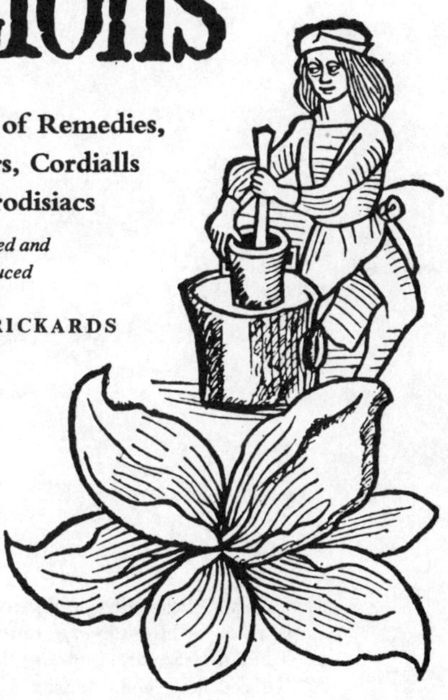

HUGH EVELYN LONDON

This edition first published
in 1968, by Hugh Evelyn Limited
9 Fitzroy Square, London, W1

Designed by Sheila Sherwen
Printed in Great Britain at The Grange Press
SBN 238 78910 1

Contents

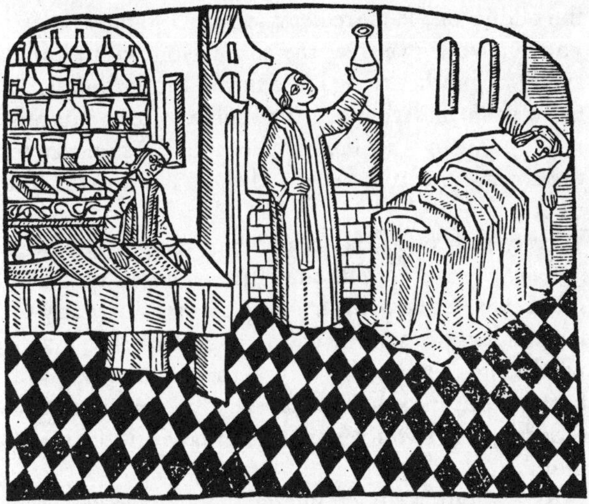

Introduction

This is a small book of optimism. Much of the material in it comes directly from the handwritten notes of our forefathers, entries in the household memorandum books that they kept, sometimes for generations, in the kitchen-table drawer or in the family treasure chest.

These 'commonplace books', as they were called, served as a storehouse of family lore and wisdom – unofficial reference books in time of need. They come down to us as insights into the personal lives of real people, centuries ago. You will notice not only the spelling, which may take a little getting used to, and the oddity of the ingredients (which also may) but as you run your eye over the entries you will become aware of another thing. As a thread throughout it all there is an underlying, irrepressible, often unjustifiable optimism – a conviction, against all evidence to the contrary, that for every ill there is a known and certain cure.

Leafing through the farmhouse pages, with here a *consumtion*, there a *fitt*, and there again an *apolletick stroak*, we see the gallantry of spirit that was ready to set juniper and gentian and *trecle* against such overwhelming odds. Here, surely, as the ancient book was brought out into the kitchen firelight, was optimism unsurpassed. It was very much a matter, it seems, of morale.

As though to underline the point there is the occasional final flourish to a prescription: *This will give ease in extreme pain and torture.* Or: *Is good for Cold stiches and Wind, Tooth Ack, pain in the Head and deafness being applyed in cotton in the ear and excellent for all bruises both externall and internall.* For failing courage, for the lengthening pangs of pessimism, what could be more heartening to the sufferer than these? Like the printed labels of encouragement that today's proprietaries provide, these built-in notes of confidence abound. Sometimes – surely most cheering of all – the note appears in a different hand as an addendum: *It is proved.*

If these notes of recommendation were calculated to raise morale, it may also be reflected that they obliquely under-sold the rest of the remedies – the large majority that went unsung. (Or, on the contrary, did the absence of sales-talk, the strong-silent approach, have its own authority?) Whichever way the psychology worked, it was certainly a major factor. In the spells and incantations that featured in some of the remedies, the principle of suggestibility was taken to its logical conclusion. Given the right indications, the principle still works today.

Old wives' tales or not, we know that many of the remedies actually worked. The farmhouse pharmacopoeia was not just magic and spells. The staple ingredients of these early therapies are with us still.

Before we smile too broadly at their caraway, juniper, coriander, cardamoms and senna pods, we must remind ourselves that it was only 30 years ago that the doctor's bag contained barely half a dozen specific remedies – actual cures for diseases. All the rest were palliatives, sedatives, stimulants, tonics and fever-reducers – not cures, but aids to the patient in his own fight against disease. And more than half the substances that the general practitioner prescribed in the earlier years of the twentieth century had been the daily stock-in-trade of the ancients and of the Arabic-speaking physicians of the Middle Ages. Two-thirds of these medicines of the 1930s had been known to the ancient Greeks. The pharmacists of only yesterday were compounding, as Lord Ritchie-Calder reminds us 'medicaments mentioned in the Egyptian papyri, including alloes, caraway, coriander, dill, fennel, juniper, mint, myrrh and turpentine, and salts of copper and lead'. To this twentieth-century list the

Assyrians had contributed almond oil, galbanum and liquorice, and the Indians, from their remote past, had given cardamoms, senna pods and jimson weed.

Much has happened in medicine since the 1930s, but we are not so far removed from the *correandry* and *turpitine* as at first appears.

We are not so far, either, from many of the ills they sought to cure. Hart burn, tooth-ack, diziniss in the Head, disgestion, lowness of spirits, the gripe, grumbling in the guts and a wambling stomack – these have a familiar, almost a friendly, ring. And it is only their spelling that clouds our instant recognition of diseases like *Jonders*. Spelling too confuses us in some of the ingredients; we are at first dismayed by *gensham*, by *rubub*, *sinomon* and *salvelatterny*, but they solve themselves by saying them aloud. (How would you have spelt *sal volatile* in 1770?)

Whatever their sources, commonplace note or printed handbook, the entries show unending versatility of intake. There is scarcely a substance known to man, it seems, that has not featured in some capacity or other as a contributor to his well-being. Palatable or not, mentionable or not, all is grist to the pestle and mortar. And into the farmhouse pot has gone a wild assortment of undesirables – perhaps none more odd than that recommended by Mrs Hale for her burn ointment (page 16), with geese, sheep, hens and pigeons all contributing. Even Mrs Beeton (beyond criticism on any score) has an odd ingredient in a recipe for a scorch-mark remover. This kind of thing crops up oftener than you might think.

Of the many date lines in history on which we can congratulate ourselves for our absence, most notable are London 1625, 1636 and 1665. Optimistic indeed – optimistic to the point of tears – are the plague-preventers – the *spunge soaked in herbe of grace water*, the *hande-full of worme-wood* and the *18 pennyweight of garlick*. The Plagues brought nostrums untold, all of them absolutely useless. Perhaps there has never been a more poignant list of remedies anywhere else in the world, before or since. Even *the Kings Majesty's excellent Receipt* of nutmegs, treacle and Angelican water, availed Londoners nothing. The best advice (which the king himself took) was to get out of town. For those who stayed, there were nutmegs, garlic – and the raised morale that comes from reading recipes for remedies. Who knows – perhaps even against the Plague psychology worked.

For the department of aphrodisiacs we turn to the Kama Sutra and points east. Here again, optimism riotously prevails. With the same tortuous complexity and variety of ingredient as the aches and pains department, aphrodisiacs promise everything. Most men say that they promise more than they perform; some are not so sure. Here again there is scarcely a substance whose contribution has not been confidently invoked. But here again we are obliged to conclude that psychology is at work. Biologists tell us that it is really a matter of contented nourishment, that there is little loving done on emptiness, that a little of what you fancy is what you really need. Like food. Many a man has gone fruitlessly through exotic menus – only to find on subsequent unscheduled occasions that he prospered best on steak and chips. But, for all that, you may care to make a note of the cardamom seeds, the sandalwood and the oil of jasmine.

This is a small book of optimism. It is a distillation of Man's hope – to break beyond his cage, to extend his bounds of possibility; to better himself, to improve himself, to cure himself, to save himself. From a hickup to an epidemick, from buggs to the bite of a mad dog, from frigidity to infidelity, from bad smells to freckles – whatever ailed you, here was hope. And you never know; like the caraway and coriander, there might be something in it . . .

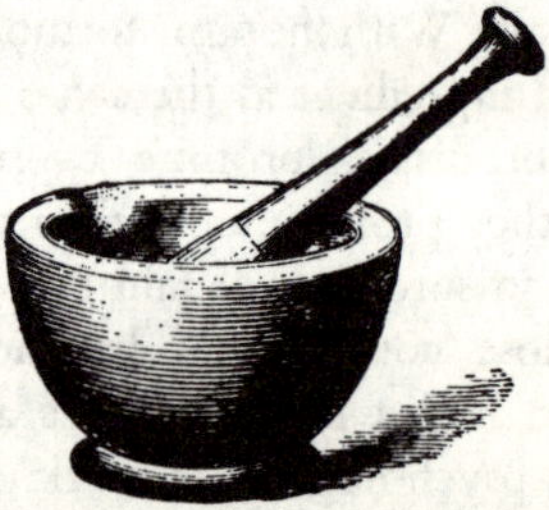

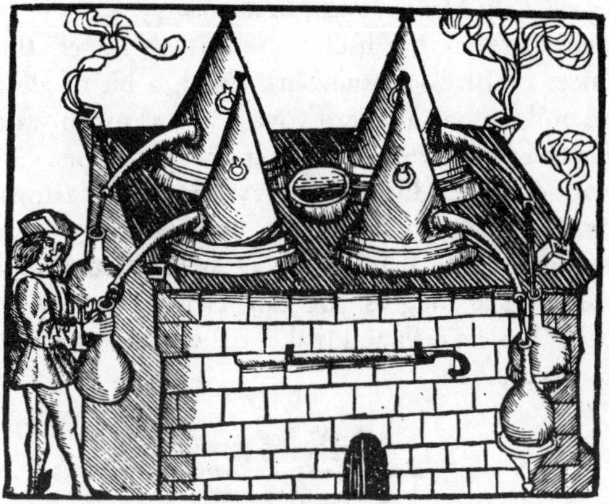

Medicinal

For a Blow, or hurt in the Eye

Beat the leaves of Eyebright with a rotten Apple, and lay it on the Eye as a poultis. Repeat it as it grows dry. The juice of the Eyebright is best.

For a Looseness, and Gripes

Infuse a pound of Poppies in halfe a pint of Spirit of Wine. Take a large Spoonfull of this liquor, with six drops of Oil of Juniper, in a Glass of Black Cherry water, sweetened with double refined sugar powdered, and mixt well with the Oil, or the Oil will swim at the top. This will give ease in extream pain, and torture.

A good daily Mouth Water, in the Scurvy

Take halfe an handfull of red Rose leaves, three ounces of Black-thorne Bark shred, a bit of allom, and boil these in a pint of Claret, and as much water, till a third is wasted, then put in the peel of one Cevil Orange, an handfull of Scurvy Grass, and as much powdered Myrrh as will go on a shilling, stir all together, and let it boil up, then strain it, and hold a mouthfull as long as you can, twice a day. It also fastens loose Teeth and makes the Gums grow up to the Teeth.

An Extraordinary Remedy for Lunacy

Take ground Ivy three large handfulls shred small, boil it in two quarts of white wine, till two parts in three be consumed, strain and add it to five ounces of the best Sallad Oil, boil it up to an ointment, let the Patient's head be shaved, then rub and chafe it with the ointment made warm; Then take fresh herbs bruised and applied Plaister ways, tying it on the top of the head very hard. Repeat this every other day, ten or twelve times, give the patient three spoonfull of the juice of Ground Ivy every morning fasting, in a glass of beer, for the first ten days.

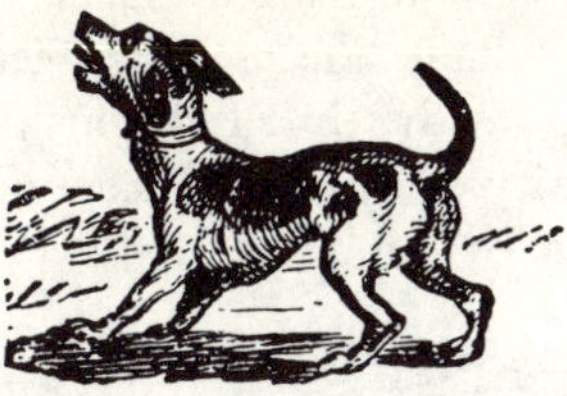

The French Method for the bite of a Mad Dog

Take the leaves of Rue, Vervin, the lesser Sage, Plantane, Polypody, Common Wormwood, Mint, Motherwort, Balm, Betony, St. Johns Wort of each an equall quantity; Gather these in June, tie them up in little bundles, which are to be wrapt up in papers, and hung up in the air where it is shady, and when wanted pound them so fine as to sift through a silk or Lawn srieve. The dose is from two to three drams of this powder, with halfe a dram of the powder of Vipers flesh, in a glass of good white wine, in a morning fasting, for two and fifty days together; if the bite is near the head or face, you must double the dose; In this you are cautioned against washing the wound with water, which contradicts our English practice of going to the sea for that purpose. However since it is necessary to cleanse off the foam or blood, Camphirated Spirit, or Spirit of Myrrh is better to wash with. Tho no remedy is so sure as the liver of the Dog, dry and powder it immediately and give from three to six ounces of it in wine, syrup, or any other way, and depend on it it is the best medicine yet discovered for that sad malady. Take the quantity in twenty four hours if possible.

Mrs Hales Ointment for Burns or Scalds

Take of Goose dung, Sheeps dung, Hens dung, and Pidgeons dung (at the time Pidgeons go a pecking) an equal quantity of each, boyl them up together in fresh hogs Lard, or Lamb suet.

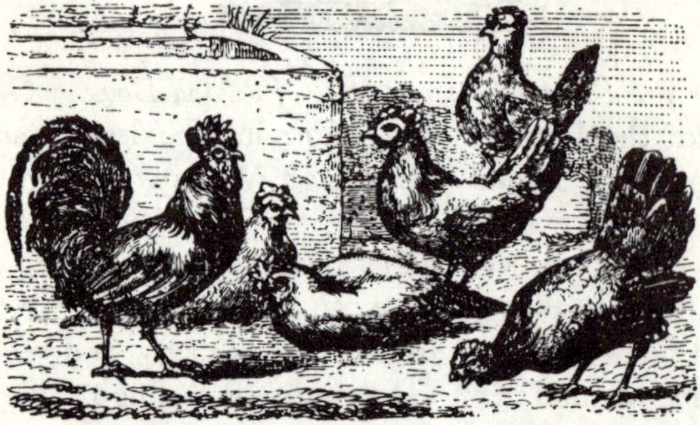

An Excellent Powder for Convulsion Fitts

Take two drams of Piony roots, misletoe of the Oak one dram, prepared Pearl, white Amber prepared, and prepared Coral, of each half a dram; Bezoar two grains, and five leaves of gold; Make all these into a very fine powder, and give as much of it as will lie upon a threepence, to a Child of a month old, and proportionable to a bigger. Mix it up with a spoonfull of Black Cherry water which sweeten with the Syrrup Black Cherries. Take it at every change of the Moon, to prevent returns, three days together.

An Ointment which is a certain cure for any Scabs, Pimples, or old Inveterate Itch

Take a quarter of an ounce of red Precipitate. Grind it on a Marble stone till it is as fine as the flower of Brimstone, then mix it up with an ounce of flower of Brimstone, and work both up with three ounces of Butter without salt as it comes from the Churn; mix it very well, and anoint the place, very thin, with the ointment. It is not the nature of it to check, but to draw out the distemper, and in a week or ten days confinement it will make an absolute cure.

For the Bite of a mad Dog

Take four ounces of Rue, four ounces of London Treacle, four spoonfull of scraped Pewter, and four ounces of Garlick, and boil all in a bottle of stale strong Ale, strain it, and let that which is thick be applyed to the wound and take nine spoonfull of the clear for nine days together.

A Posset Drink, taken before the Ague fitt

Pour a Gallon of clear Posset drink upon four large handfull of Angelica shred small, let it infuse till it is very strong; let the person if possible drink all, that the stomack may be perfectly clear, and go into a warm bed when the Vomet hath done working. Cover your selfe close, and try to sweat.

A good Epidemick Water

Take, Rue, Rosemary, Pimpernel, Balm, Dragon, Marygold flowers and leaves, Mint and Angelica, of each two handfull, also the roots of Elerampane, Piony, Master Wort, of each one pound, Gentian, Tormentill and Virginia Snake Wood, of each four ounces, Saffron one ounce; infuse all these when shred in two quarts of white wine, one quart of water and one quart of French Brandy distilled. Use it in any malignant Distemper.

For a Surfeit

Boil a handfull of fresh or dryed Poppies in Ale, with an ounce of bruised Carraway seeds, sweeten it and drink a large draught. And if the stomack is so sick as to discharge it, repeat it again, till it doth stay in the stomach, and sleep on it.

For a convulsive Colick

Take yellow transparent Amber, grossly powdered, Ginger minted, and fill a Pipe, and smoak three or four, while in pain, and always going to rest.

To prevent the Nail growing into the Toe

If the Nail be hard and thick, and grows into the Toe, take a piece of broken glass, and scrape it very thin on the top. Do this when ever you cut your Nails, and by constant use it makes the corners fly up, and grow more flat.

Syrup of Snailes

You must prick your Snails, and strew sugar upon them and hang them up in a bag, and catch the droppings. Drink a draught thrice a day.

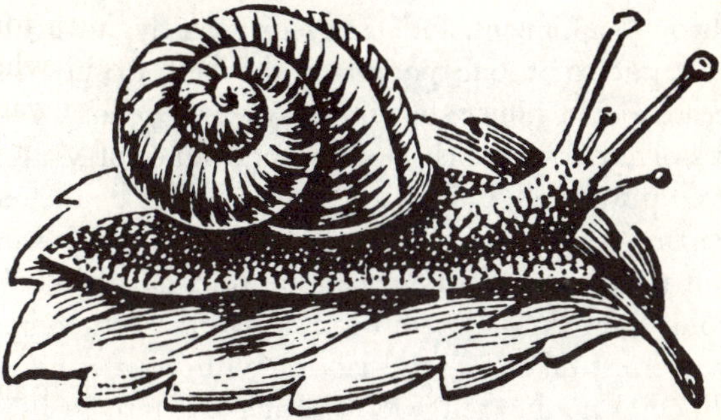

To cure the Itch, tho of long Continuance

Take eight or nine spoonfull of Conduit water, and two or three spoonfull of common Treacle, three or four spoonfull of white wine Vinegar, enough to make it sharp, stir it well together and let the party take two spoonfull the first morning, four the second and eight the third, for this brings the Itch thoroughly out; Then at night anoint the party with flower of Brimstone, beaten Ginger and fresh Butter, this you must do for three nights together. Be sure you put on clean sheets and all clean Linnen on your selfe, well aired before you begin to anoint. And after you have anointed three nights, wash all over, in warm water, and put on clean Linnen well aired again. This hathe cured the Itch of seven years standing.

To make the Salve Gratia Dei, which is to be made about Midsummer

Take Vervain, Betony and Pimpernell, of each one handfull, stamp them, and boil them in three quarts of white Wine, till halfe be consumed, then strain it through a Linnen Cloth, and set it over the fire again, and put to it one pound of the best Rosin, well beaten, four ounces of virgin Wax, or yellow Wax dissolved in womans Milk, and one ounce of Mastick well powdered, boil all in the wine, till it be melted, stirring it well and fast, then take it from the fire and put to it a pound of Turpentine, stirring it till it be cold, then the salve will rise above the rest, which you must take out, and labour with your hands as shoemakers do their wax, and make it into Rolls.

It is good for all sorts of wounds, new and old, it cleanses and heales, eateth of dead flesh and generateth new, it mollifies Boils, draws out Thorns, breaks Imposthumes, is good in the Canker and a fistula and bruises on the sinews, St. Anthony fire, and it asswageth great swellings.

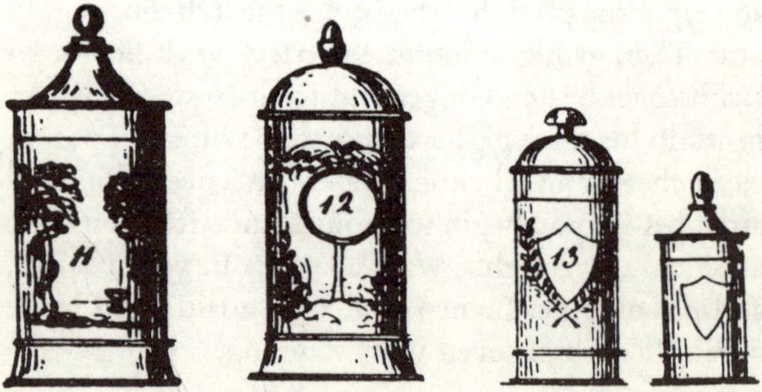

To cure Deafness and noise in the head

Put your own urine into a pewter dish, and cover it with another, then put some Coals under and when it is hot, brush off the clear water that hangs on the upper dish with a feather, and drop it into the Ear; This hath done great cures.

For the Jaundice

To four pounds of the husks of Wallnuts, put half a pound of Wormseed, and as much flower of Brimstone. Draw it off in a cold still, and let a Tea cup full be taken every morning for a month. This is an excellent Medicine for Jaundice, and hath done great cures.

A very good Powder for a Dizziness in the Head and to prevent Apoplectick Fitts

Take the seeds and roots of single Piony, of each a like quantity, dry and beat them severally into a fine powder, take the weight in Nutmeg, which you must beat and dry, and beat again; mix fine sifted sugar with this and take as much as will lie on a shilling every morning for a month constantly.

A Powder to stop the Hickup

Put as much Dill food, finely powdered, as will lie upon a shilling, into two spoonfull of Syrup of Black Cherries, and take it presently. It will stop them in man, woman or Child.

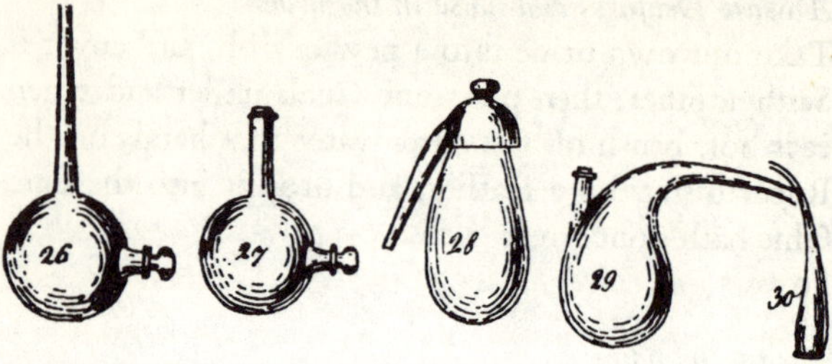

A very good Snail Water for a Consumption

Take half a peck of shell snails, wipe them, and bruise them shells and all in a Mortar; put to them a gallon of New Milk; as also Hysop and Burrage, of each one handfull, Figs, Raisons in the sun stoned, and Dates of each a quartar a pound, with two large Nutmegs. Put them to the Milk, and distill it with a quick fire in a cold still. This will yeild near four wine quarts of water very good: You must put two ounces of white sugar Candy into each bottle, and let the water drop on it, stir the herbs some times while it distills. Take five spoonfull at a time, first and last, and at four in the afternoon.

A good Cordiall Water for the Spleen

Take four ounces of Hartshorne, one ounce of Cardamoms, one ounce of Cinnamon, one ounce of Saffron, two handfull of Red sage, as much Balm; Steep these for twenty four hours in two quarts of sack, or as much good Brandy which you please. Distill it in a cold still as quick as you can, and let it drop on four ounces of sugar Candy. Drink of this when low spirited.

A Milk Water for the Evill
Take roots of Daisies, Burdock, Guajarum, Sassafras, Sarsaparilla, China, Formentill and Hounds tongue, each two ounces; Selendine, Yarrow, Plantain, Herb Robert, Agremony, Speedwell, Ground Ivy and Cinquefoil, of each a large handfull, Archangel flowers one pint; Sweet Sorrell and Coriander seeds of each one ounce. Shred and bruise all, and put them in a gallon of milk, draw off as much as runs good, and drink daily a quarter of a pint every four hours. And into each draught squeeze the juice of a small spoonfull of Millepedes.

— *Receipts in Physick, Surgery, etc.*
(*Commonplace Book of Elizabeth Plowman*) 1731

Mrs Sherlock's recept for a pain in ye head
2 ounses of Rubbarb leaves sliced, i ounse of Jeusit's bark in powder, 2 ounses of sugar candy, 2 drams of Juniper Berris, Sinamon & nutmeg of each a dram: a Quart of strong wine infuse it in.

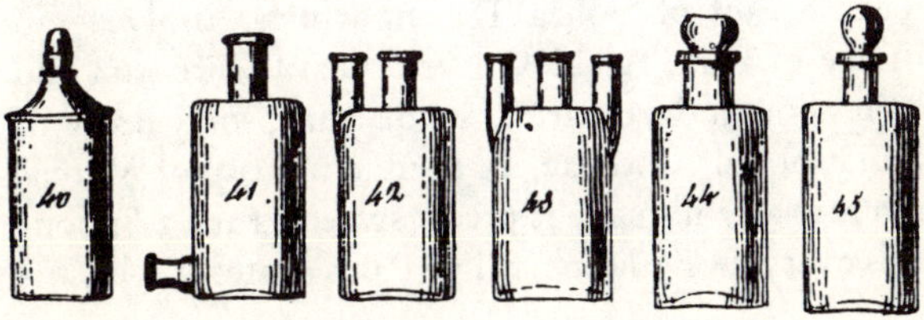

How to make a Cordiall Broath

Take 3 Sheeps Hinges with the wool on their heads: 3 dozen of Sheep Trotters: 2 Bullocks Livers, with half a peck of Oat meal. Boyl all these in a Caldron 2 hours, then strain the Broath through a hair sackcloth, and let it cool. The use of it is to appease grumbling in the Guts, or a wambling stomack, by drinking one Pot at a time and eating the meat after it. This will preserve you from hunger and wind in the Stomack, using it but once in 2 hours.

For Consumption

Take 30 garden snails & 30 Earth worms of middling sise, bruise ye snails & wash them & ye worms in fair waters, cut ye worms in pieces. Boil these in a quart of Spring water to a pint. Pour it boiling on 2 ounses of Candied Eringo root sliced thin. When it is cold strain it thro a fine flannel bag. Take a quarter of a pint of it warm, with an equal Quantity of Cows' milk till well, at twilight.

— quoted in *A Cordiall Water*, M. F. K. Fisher

For the Cholick & Gravel

Take a Pint of Bohea Tea, in which dissolve ½ an ounce of Gum Arabick over a Gentle Fire, thn add to it about a third part of white wine, forty drops of Spirit of Sal Amoniac, & as much Syrup of Marchmallow as will make it pretty sweett. Take 3 Spoonfuls every 2 or 3 hours, till ye Pains abate.

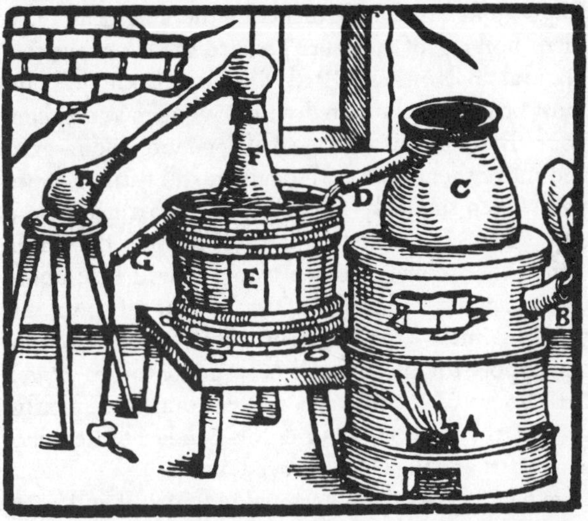

An Excellent Balsam of Dr Baptista Navrella

1st: New Yellow Bees Wax 8oz, Dragons blood ½oz; Sweet Marjoram, Bay Leaves, tops of Rosemary of each an handfull. Put the above into an earthen pot well glazed. *2nd:* Oyl Capivi 2oz, Liquid Storax 6oz, VeniceTurpentine 4oz, Balsam hipericum 2oz, Olive Oyl a pound, Rose Water 12oz, Spring Water a pound, Plantain Water 12oz, Old Mallaga Sack 2 pounds – put these into a large pot well glazed. *3rd:* Natural Balsam of Peru 2oz, Red Sanders ½oz.

To make it: Take a pot that contains a quart, another that contains 8 quarts, set both at the same time over a moderate fire, put into the smallest pot the Wax and other first ingredients. Into the larger pot put the Oyl

Capivi and other ingredients of the 2nd Class. Let them boil a $\frac{1}{4}$ of an hour. Then to the latter put the Natural Balsam and Red Sanders. Both Vessells must be constantly stirred with a wooden stick, then pour the Contents of the small pot into the larger, and make them boil well together, still stirring them well. Then suddenly cast the whole substance into a clean Napkin, straining it well before the Fire. When the strained Balsam is cold it will Dry upon the water the Colour of a Brick. Take of the solid part and melt it over a gentle Fire and put it into Galleypots for use. It will keep good for 20 years. NB your Wax must be shaved thin and gently melted, the Dragon blood & Red Sanders beaten fine each apart and the Herbs minced small.

Directions to Use it: If a deep wound, melt it and pour it into the wound with a Syringe or quill taking care not to scald. If not deep apply with a Feather or Cotton. Anoint well about the wound, every Dressing wash the part with warm wine or Vinager & Water mixed. If a Bruise or swelling apply spread like a Plaster. If for Gout, Siatica or Cholic, anoint the place well and happly as a Plaister keeping the Patient warm.

The Virtues: It is good against all accidents especially Siatica. Cold stiches & all fresh wounds may be cured by it. If first applied in 5 or 6 days leaves no scar. Is good against the Gout proceeding from Cold. Should be taken inwardly the quantity of a nutmeg going to Bed, and the stomach & Belly anointed with it. Is good for hard Corns, against all swellings and burns of Fire, Water or Gunpowder, against poison as the Bite of Serpents or Scorpions by anointing the part and taking inwardly an ounce in warm milk. For all surfeits by taking an oz inwardly warm going to bed and sweating; for spitting of blood and all Fluxes by taking the quantity of a large Nuttmeg going to bed. If bad repeat once in the day between breakfast and dinner or morning fasting. It creates appetite and Expells Wind, Draws thorns & Splinters of Bones out of the flesh & never heals but from the bottom of the wound. Is good for Cold stiches and Wind, Tooth Ack, pain in the Head and deafness being applyed in Cotton in the Ear and excellent for all bruises both externall and internall.

— *Commonplace Book, circa* 1750

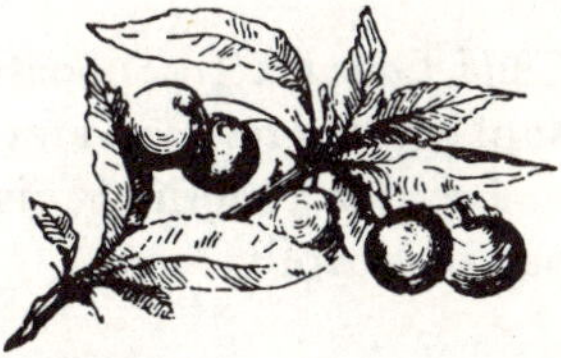

Pain in the Head
Boil Black Currin leaves or twigs in Old Milk, and put it into a Narrow topt pot and put a towel over it and let the shthem go up your Nose, into your Mouth and Ears. or horse Redish is good to smell on, or applyd to the Fore head or spt: of wine & hartshorn for a pain, but if an Umour apply Allum & Coperas water.

Waters for all sorts of wounds
Allum water, Copperas water, or Vitrol water, or Lime water, or Vinegar, or Chamberly, or Spts: of Whine or Brandy, to wash all fresh wounds make them Milk warm when you make use of them – When you use the Drying water for a sore if you think it is to sharpe do a plaster on first and then a rag on that Done round the edges in the water.

For Inflamation in the Eyes
Take Roman Vitrol, & Bole Armoniack of each 1oz, Camfer ¼oz, pounder them togather, and put ½oz of this powder into two pints of Boiling Water, stir it well about then take it off the fire and let it settle, and Decant off what is clear – You may ad a little roach Allum if you think proper.

Physick for a Child, Give it a TeaSpoonfull at a time of Goulden Spts: of Scurvegress – and for Worms, after chiwing a little Bread in a Morning, give them a little Brandy or Spts: of Vitroll.

Eyes Juist of the inner Bark of Willow, or Raw Veal applyd to it.

A Dye Drink for *apollettick Stroke* Gensham Root, Juniper Beries, Rubub, Sentuary, Mixt with the best Holland Gin, and water which is opening of water vessels and warming to the Stomack.

Tinture of Gum Goacum $1\frac{1}{2}$ Tea Spoonful in Wine or Water for the *Rhumatism.*

For Bad Breast, Cool drawn Linseed Oyl and Campherated Spts: of Whine apply'd before & after lying in.

A Leg that swells & Umoury, apply the juist of Salladine to it.

A Setfast in a Leg mix Vitrol and Greas togather to eat it out.

Rum & New-milk for a *Caugh.*

A Receit for those *Inclining to Consumtion,* Conserve of Roses $\frac{1}{2}$oz, Balsam, $\frac{1}{2}$oz, Armicompanum Powder $\frac{1}{4}$oz, Forty Drops of Balsom of peru, and a few drops of Spts of Sulfer. And take about the sise of a common nutmeg, every morning before Breckfst Drinking $\frac{1}{2}$ a pint of Tea after it mixt with a Tablespoonfull of the best Brandy And to Abstain from food that create fleam.

Crush on the Body that affects Inwardly – Drink Tent wine and Black Bear.

For a Bad Hand to gather it to a Head, Milk and Parkpale Bark, or Boild Turnip.

For the Ashma
Gunpowder and Brimston brused fine & Mixt with Tracle into a Ball or Stiff paste & take a little at Pleasure.

For Stranguary, Burn Common Black Flint till white through, then bruse it very fine pass it thro a Sirge and take what will lie on a shilling in white wine or parsely Tea at a time. Any may take it.

By John Tomson Dr. – *Diziniss in the Head*. Take Lillies of the Valley 2 Bay leaves a little of the best Tobacco Make all into snuff and take when troubled.

Hart Burn, Take Liver wort a small Quantity Boil it in small bear Drink a large TeaCup full· when you have the Hartburn.

Fainting. Old white KidneaBeans or the Black spotted, Dry'd and powdr'd take as much as will lie on a shilling in a Glass of white wine when Fainting.

Stomach, take Green Bay leaves a large handfull Dry'd and Powdr'd and mixt with Honey as an Electuary Take in a Morning 2 Teaspoonfulls and same at evening.

Take Salvalatteny dropt on lump Sugar 20 or 30 drops or more for *Sore throte* or *pain at Stomack*.
or its good for Tooth Ach. (tried)

For the Jaundice proved
Take one handfull of wormwood one
of horound one of sheep's dung boil
the same in one quart of water til
it becomes one pint strain through a cloth
the same boil the liquor in 2 pints of
ale for one Minute when cold add one
small teacupfull of Rum —

Varnish for Hatt Case
1 oz of spirits of Wine
½ — of Black sealwax
½ pennyworth of isinglass

Take 1 oz or 2 if dried marygold flowers &
and boil them in 3 pints of ale til reduce
to 1 pint add ¼ lb treacle to make a Cow drense
after calving

Tooth Ach. Spts. of Salts and water of equal Quantity mix togather & put to the tooth in a bit of Lint.

Strain in the Back, Balsom of Sulfer 1oz, Oyl of Anneseeds ¼oz, mix togather and Drop 40 Drops to some sugar and take inwardly.

Inflamation, Juist of Salladine, House leek, and Cream.

Proud Flesh in a Wound or to open a hole more, put in a little Red presipitr which I suppose is not so poisness as others.

For *Nose Bleeding*, Nettle Juist a Tea Cupfull at a Time.

Breaking out of Scabs. Rub them with HouseLeek and Cream.

Stich in the Side or windy Complaint take a little Gin and water and if Bad Blood them.

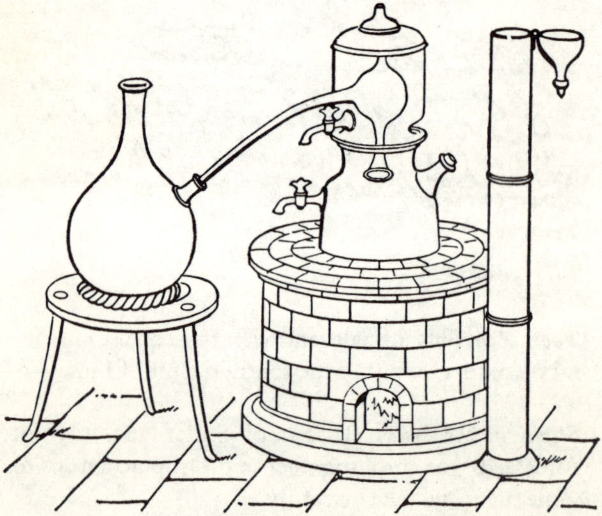

Frosty Feet, that Iches much rub them with Spts: of Vitrol or Salt peeter.

Swelling in the foot that come by itself make a poultis of white Bread and Milk & white Lilly root afterward do a little Drying water to it & they be full of Umours give them some physick.

For Sore Throat, Suck Salt peeter or Saltprunellow. or Blister and physick. or Gargle Yr throat with Hartshorn & water prity Strong.

To make physick for persons full of *Umours,* weigh by a half Guinea weight some Gollop & divide it in Three doses, with equal Quantity of Cream of Tarter. And add a little Ginger to keep it from making you sick.

For a Disgestian – 1oz of perruvian Bark ½oz of Gensham Root ½oz of Correandry seed ½oz of Orange pill dry'd powdered all togather and infused in 1 Quart of French Brandy Take a Wine Glass in a Morning & about eleven oClock – Dr. Beaucan.

For a Glister take one handfull of Cammomile flowers & half an oz of Anneseeds boil them for about ten minutes in 3 parts of a pint of water, and then strain them off and add two Table spoonfull of Oil and half a Spoonfull of Sugar. to be repeated as Need require.

Gentle physick half an Ounce of Senna half a pint of Boiling Water, Quarter of an Ounce of Correandery Seeds, infuse them for the space of an hour in a close Vessel, then disolve 1 ounce of the best Manna in it and strain of the Liquors add to the straind Liquor two Table Spoonfull of Tinture of Senna. Three Tablespoonfulls for a dose – G. Frith.

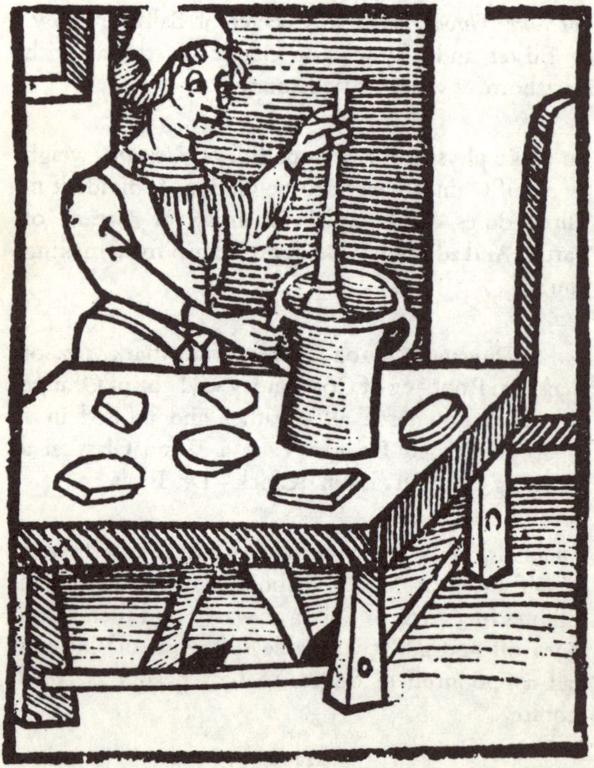

For a Running Eye or a Speck in it take the White of an Egg lay it on a plate and rub it about with a lump of Allum till it come like an ointment, and bind it on the Eye.

1oz of Salts, & 1oz or 3 pen: of the Tincture of Seany Make 2 doces of good physic. good for *inward pain.*

For a Caugh or Could Take 4 Ounces of Candy Sirup 1 Ounce of Candy Sirup 1 Ounce of Spyrmisiti ¾ of an Ounce of Saltpeter.

For the Piles 1oz of Sinomon Boild in 1 pint of Water till it come to Gill taken at Discretion. Or Pills of Pitch are supposed Cure.

For a person that appears to have over much Blood and it appears improper to Blood them. let them take a Table spoonfull of Salt repeatedly & Drink Tarr Water.

For Inward Complaint or Lowness of Spts: ½oz of Nitre Adulser, & ½oz of Compound Spts of Lavinder take about a Teaspoonfull at a time.

For a Swelled Hand That's full of pain take Cammomile, Milk & Bread for pultice, to take pain out, then Apply Wormwood, Salt, & Vinegar.

For the Eyes, take White of an Egg & rub it with a Lump of Allum upon a Pewter plate till it come to a Curd for an inflamation may bind it on the eye.

For the Shakg Jonders, Take Castile Soap & the Best Rubub equal quantity & make into Pills the size of Marrow pea & take 3 for 3 times a Day.

Oil of Tarr for the *Tooth Ach*.

Drink for Fever – Putrid or Scarlet – known to be good Take 2 or 3 Ounce of Comn Barley Boil it till it Burst in abt 2 Quarts of water then pour it of & add to it 2 or 3 Spooful of Juce of Hoise-leek, & the same Quantity of Vinegar Sweetned with Honey to take as Comn Drink. Barm or New Ale with Barm Give to throw out the Eruption Barm was Recommended in Newspaper for putrid fever.

For Spitting of Blood & Corruption. Get Cup Moss of an Oak Tree or Pales & dry it in an oven & powder it & pass it thro some gauze & mix abt a Teacup full in abt $\frac{1}{2}$lb Trecle & take it Morning & Night or any time when troubled with the Caugh.

Person
For a person that has a *pain in his back* that has come by a hurt & afterward caused by çold. In about ½ a TeaCupfull of Tracle mix abt ½ an Ounce of Sulphur of Vivum & take 2 or 3 Tea Spoonfulls of it as you find Occation.

For *Shortness of Breath* when they cannot sleep at Nights Tak a Tea spoonfull of Sirrup of Squils n a little Water at Bedtime, (its Rather a Binding effect.).
Jno Eyre tried it.

Medicin for *Scurvey* Take 2 oz of Flower of Brimstone Boil it in 2 Qrts of Water to 3 pints then Clear it off put it into a Bottle. Take 1 wine Glass full every Morning while done. then take Saltpeeter as much as will lay on Sixpence every Morng for a week in water, then Boil the Old Brimston over again and take it as before.

Salvelatterny & Spts of Lavinder for *lowness of Spirits.*

For a *Raw place that wants healing* – Sweet Oil and white Lead or Brimstone.

To take the pain out of a *Crush* – Apply stewed Cammomile & linceed Oil.

Stoppage of water, Marchmellow & parseley Roots, & Salts of prunellow & Dandelion.

A Sore Throte, apply sweet Eating Oil and Artshorn to it & Stocking foot at Night Suck Salt peeter.

Dye Drink for a *Nervous Complaint or lowness of Spirits*, Ground Ivey, wormwood, Camomile Flowers, water Trafehole, scurvGrass, Boam, Erbegrass, HorseRedish, 1 Pound of Coarse sugar 2 Gallons of your best liquor and boild togather No hops.

Erbegrass good *for fits in Children*

— *Commonplace Book, circa* 1770

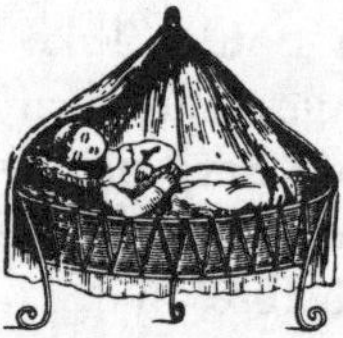

For a Cough; When you are going to bed, drink Brandy Treacle and sallad oil mixed.

For the Itch
Take Frankincense and beat it small, and mingle it with oil of Bays and therewith anoint all over.

For the Lice
Take Oblibnum mixed with as much Brawns Grease beat the Oblibnum first into fine powder and boyled together make an ointment.

For the Jaundice proved
Take one handfull of wormwood one of horound one of sheep's dung boil the same in quart of water till it becomes one pint strain through a cloth the same boil the liquor in 2 pints of ale for one Minute when cold add one small teacupfull of Rum.

Remedy for the Itch. For a large Family Take one quart of Rum one oz of Black peper powdred and Defuse them togather for 24 Hours Rub the parts affected Approved.

Gas tar and yellow Oker make an excellent green Paint.

Cholera Morbus

Tincture of Huxham		6	Drams
Do	Rhubarb	4	Do
Do	Opium	2	Do
Do	Benjamin	2	Do
Elexir of Vitriol		4	Do
		18	

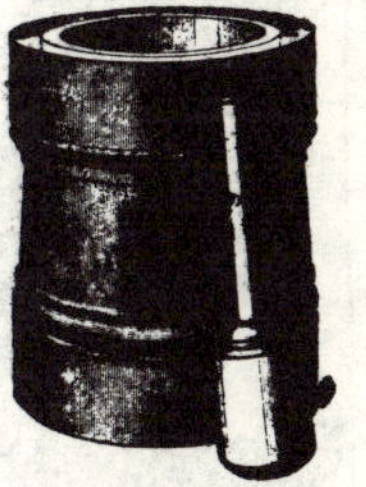

A Teaspoonful or two, three or four times a day, if very bad three teaspoonsful at a time.

Cure for Spasmodic Cholera take 3 Drops of Croton Oil on a little sugar.

from the Gazette of Yorkshire

For Burn or Scald apply soft soap immeadiately.

For a week Constitution
Take a large handful of Bean Grass and boil in three quarts of water until reduced to two, then strain the herbs from the liquor and put in a Gill of Honey and boil it again till reduced to three Pints. Two Table spoonsful to be taken every morning fasting and a Tea Spoonfull of Syrup of Violets immediately after.

– *Jane Foley's Commonplace Book*

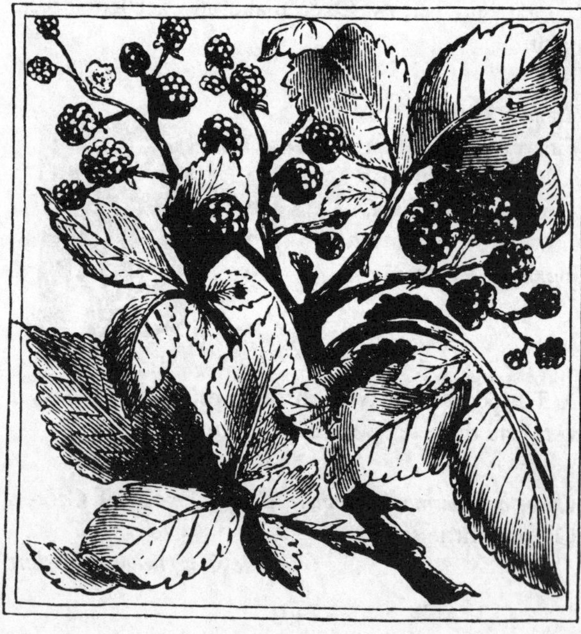

Remedy for haemorrhoids

Take finely powdered slate; mix it with a little oil or butter to make an ointment. Apply it the haemorrhoids.

Remedy for burns

Take lime water and walnut oil, equal parts; beat them together and anoint the burns.

Remedy for smallpox spots

Take the oldest kitchen fat that you can and mix it with oats; set fire to the oats and let the drops of grease that come from it to fall on the surface of frshly-drawn well water. Collect these and apply them to the face after the breaking of the pimples.

Remedy against inflammation of the eyes caused by smallpox

Take equal parts of rose-water and plantain-water, with just a little saffron, to bathe the bad eyes. If the eyes are runny, add a little white vitriol.

Remedy against chilblains

Take some old kitchen fat, rub it in the hands, taking care to keep them gloved at night.

Remedy for corns

Take some diapalme, make a little ball with it and in it a little natural yellow arsenic; leave long enough to give the arsenic time to eat away the corn.

Remedy for callouses
They must be rubbed with a little juice of celandine, and be careful to cut them from time to time towards the centre.

Remedy for fits
Take, while it is in flower, the plant called Mouron with the blue flowers, dry it between papers, & reduce it to a powder, of which you will give a demi-gros twice a day for a fortnight. It is said that this plant even cures those who have already had fits.

Remedy for tooth-ache
Take one ounce of piretre root. After bruising and crushing, pour over it five ounces of wine-spirit; you will get from this a sour red tincture, of which put a small spoonful in the mouth & leave it until the mouth fills up with saliva. It is rare that one is obliged to repeat the remedy without having abated the pain.

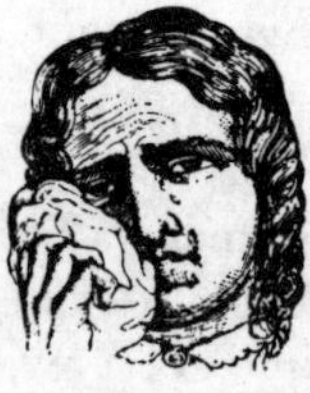

Another remedy for tooth-ache
Take a pinch of sea-salt, finely reduced to a powder, a clove & a thimbleful of gunpowder, crush them together in such a way as to form a kind of ointment. Apply it on a cloth towards the temple.

To strengthen the gums
Take two ounces of scurvy-grass spirits, fourteen ounces of brandy & a demi-gros of Red Balm; put them all together to make up a milky liquid, a spoonful to be used every morning in the mouth. Rub the gum lightly and rinse with a little water and vinegar.

Four-robbers Vinegar
Four-robbers Vinegar specially suitable for use in the country. It is of a strong odour, aromatic, mixed with garlic and camphor. It is best to choose a penetrating sort. It is used to protect oneself from the Bad Airs, sprinkling it freely on the clothes and washing the face with it. One may, before going into contagious places, rinse the mouth with the fluid; but as one may sometimes either be without it or be surprised by unexpected contagion, use a substitute either of good strong vinegar or by vinegar in which one has infused a number of knobs of garlic.

—*Economie Rustique* ou *Notions Simples et Faciles*
Published in Paris by Lottin le jeune, 1779

For Convulsions: Take cuttings of the sick person's nails, some hair from the eyebrows and a halfpenny, wrap them altogether in a cloth which has been round the patient's head and place the bundle in a gateway where four lanes meet. The first person who finds and opens it will take the disorder himself, relieving the afflicted one.

—*John Dougall* (Edinburgh)

A 'Sympathetic Ointment' to put upon a weapon that has inflicted a wound, thus healing the wound:

Take four ounces each of boar's fat and bear's fat, boil slowly for half an hour, then pour on cold water. Skim off the floating fat, rejecting that which sinks (the older the animal yielding the fat, the better). Take of powdered burnt worms, of dried boar's brain, of red sandalwood, of mummy, and of bloodstone, one ounce each. Then collect one drachm of the moss from the skull of a man who died a violent death (one who had been hanged, preferably) and had not been buried. This should be collected at the rising of the moon, and under Venus if possible, but certainly not under Mars or Saturn. With all these ingredients, keep in a closed vessel. If it becomes dry on keeping, it can be softened with a little fresh lard or virgin honey. The ointment must be prepared in the autumn.

— *Paracelcus*

For colds in the head and in case a man clears his throat heavily, take this wort, which the Romans call marrubium and also the English call horehound, seethe it in water, give it to them that clear the throat heavily; it will heal them wonderfully. For Lung disease; take this same wort seethe it in honey, give it to swallow he will be wonderfully healed.

For ache of loins and sores of the thighs take this same wort, pulegium and pepper of either alike much by weight; pound them together and when thou be in the bath smear them where it most troubleth.

— *Herbarium of Apuleius Platonicus*

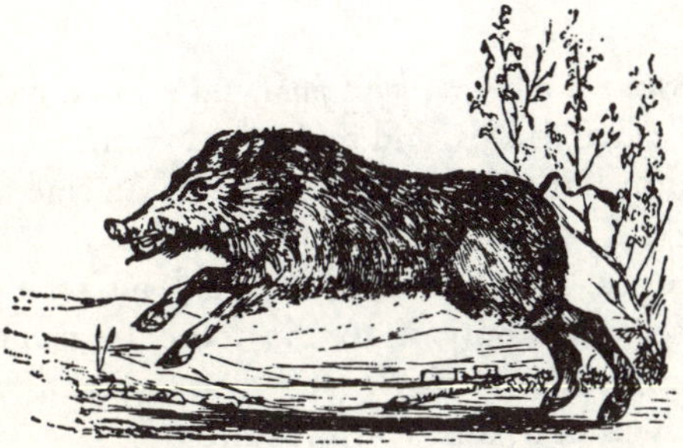

For deafness: ram's urine, eel's bile and juice of ash expressed and placed in the ears. *For punctured wound:* take the dung of a bull and apply thereto. *To induce sleep:* take poppy heads bruised in wine. For *falling sickness:* burn a goat's horn, directing the smoke against the patient. He will forthwith rise. Before he has risen from the ground, apply dog's gall upon his head and the disease will not attack him any more.

— *The Physicians of Myddfai*

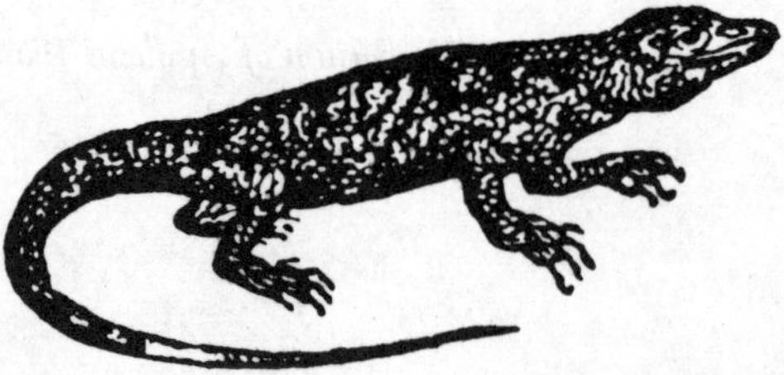

To extract a tooth without pain: take some newts, by some called lizards, and those nasty beetles which are found in ferns in the summer time. Calcine them in an iron pot and make a powder thereof. Wet the forefinger of the right hand and insert it in the powder and apply it to the tooth frequently, refraining from spitting it off, when the tooth will fall away without pain. It is proven.

For pain in the eye: take the gall of a hare, of a hen, of an eel and of a stag with fresh urine and honeysuckle leaves and then inflict a wound upon an ivy tree, mix the gum that exudeth from the ivy tree therewith, boiling it quickly and straining it through a fine linen cloth. When cold, insert a little thereof in the corner of the eye and it will be a wonder if he who makes use of it does not see stars in mid-day, in consequence of the virtues of this remedy.

For Stranguary and Stone: take the blood and skin of a hare and make a powder thereof; mix with the cyder of red-rinded apples, mead or beer and drink it with either. Let the patient drink this only. If you should wish to prove this, take a spoonful of the powder with water and put it in a hole made in an acid stone and by next day it will have certainly dissolved part of the stone.

An ointment for all kinds of aches: take gander's fat, the fat of a male cat, and red boar's fat and three drams of blue wax, water cress, wormwood, the red strawberry plant and primrose. Boil them in pure spring water and when boiled stuff a gander with them and roast them at a distance from the fire. The grease issuing from it should be carefully kept in a pot. It is a valuable ointment for all kinds of aches in a man's body and is like one that was formerly made by Hippocrates. It is proved.

— *Howel the Physician* (Wales)

Stimulating lotion
1 oz. of compound camphor liniment, mixed with 1 oz. of soap liniment, may be rubbed upon the chest with the hand in cases of chest cold, or applied on a flannel round the throat in quinsy.

Evaporating Lotion
Sal-ammoniac, ½an ounce; vinegar, 5 ozs.; rectified spirit, 5 ozs.; water, a pint. Mix together. This is a useful application in sprains and bruises, and also for the head in cases of inflamation of the brain. Rags steeped in the lotion should be kept constantly applied.

— *Mrs Beeton* 1909

Harvesters' Embrocation
Mix a cupful each of vinegar and turpentine, add a dessertspoonful of powdered camphor and an egg. Shake all together until creamy.

Roseleaf Pillow
To well-dried rose petals and sweet briar leaves add dried mint and pounded cloves. Mix well and stuff a small pillow with the mixture, to induce sleep and fragrant dreams.

— *A Calendar of Country Recipes*
Nell Heaton (Faber and Faber)

A remedy for festering sores or whitlows (1960s)
Heat a whole lemon, make a tunnel down the centre; pack this with common salt and place the affected finger within, keeping it buried in the lemon as long as possible. Repeat the treatment as needed until the ailment is cured.

To keep away mosquitoes and midges when spending evenings out-of-doors
Gather some of the aromatic herbs, such as sage, rosemary, elecampane and others, add some dry paper or dry grass, place in quite large open cans, sprinkle the herb, etc. with paraffin and ignite: the pungent smoke will clear the air of mosquitoes and kindred biting insects.

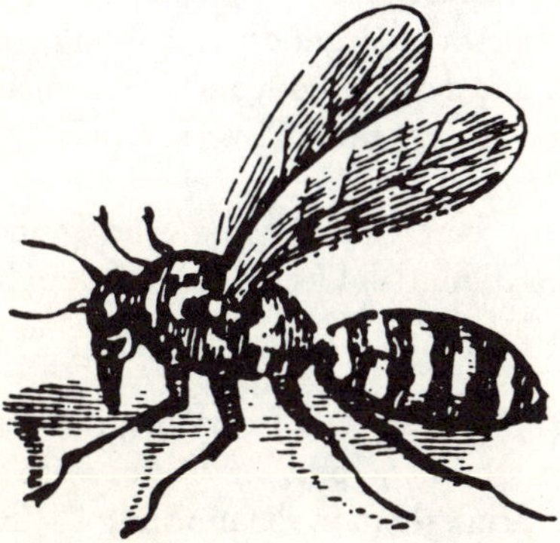

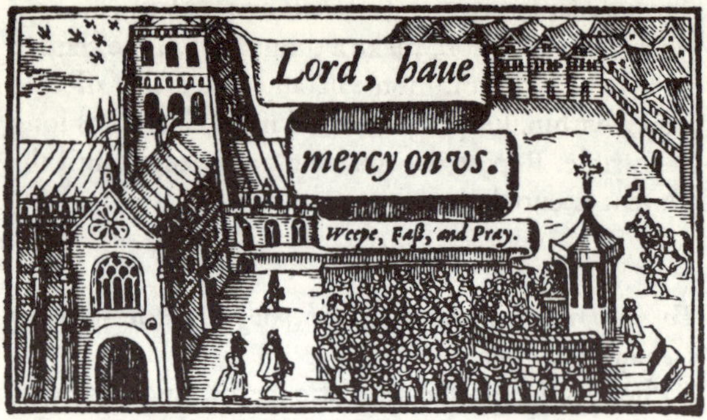

The Plague

Take white Sponge soaked in herbe of grace water, which water is thus made: Take a quart of Vinegar, halfe a pint of Rosewater, put in a hand-full of Rue, and halfe and hand-full of worme-wood, and boile it to a pint; then take and dip the Spunge in it when it is cold, and hold it to your nose when you go abroad: and this is a good Preservative.

Take of the best Cedar wood, and grate a small wooden boxe full, and let the lid be full of holes, and smell to it.

Take worme-wood, and herbe of grace, and steep them all night in a pint of beere, with a lemon sliced, and drink them in the morning fasting.

Take a Wal-nut kernell, a corne of salt, foure leaves of herbe of grace; cut all very small, and put them in a blue figge, and roast it, and fast one houre after: but use it daily.

Take a toste of bread, and spread it over with Treacle and butter, and herbe of grace eaten with it is very good.

Take Endive water a quart, Century water a pint, Ivie berries halfe an hand-full bruised. Boile these together gently a quarter of an houre, and when you take it from the fire, dissolve therein as much Treacle as a Nut, and a little Sugar, also put thereunto three spoonefuls of Vinegar. As soone as the Patient doth complaine, and Nature being yet strong, give him fasting one good draught thereof warme, and let him keepe his bed, and sweat ten houres, or lesse, as the strength of the Patient will beare. In his sweating give him now and then Ale clarified, and into every draught put two or three spoone-fuls of the decoction. When he riseth, give him some broth, not made over strong, neither with much spice: and be very careful to keep him from the ayre. This decoction thus used will either force out the Sore, or else if the Patient sweat throughly well, cure him without any Sore. And it thou find he be not greatly eased within eight houres after his sweating, the next day use the like order.

Take of cloves of garlick 18.penny weight, of fresh butter 3.ounces, of lemon the weight of a shilling, a white onion cut in pieces, a hand-full of malloes, and a hand-full of scallions; boil these in a pottell of water, and make them a poultis,.and lay to the Sore very warm. Renew it every day.

Take a hot loafe newly drawne, and lay to it, but when you take it away lay a fresh, but be sure to burie the bread after.

To aire a house, take Cedar or Juniper, Lavender and dry Bayes, and old Rosemary, put them in a pan of coals in the middle of a house.

Take the same with Rose-water and Vinegar, & lay the Bed upon an hurdell, or frame of a table, with staves to stay it up, and set two or three Chafing dishes under: & this is an excellent receit to air clothes. London 1636

The Kings Majesty's excellent Receipt for the Plague
Take half an ounce of nutmegs and add a penny-worth of treacle, and a quart of the best Angelican water, beat them all together, put it over the fire a little. Take it always warm, both morning and evening. London 1665

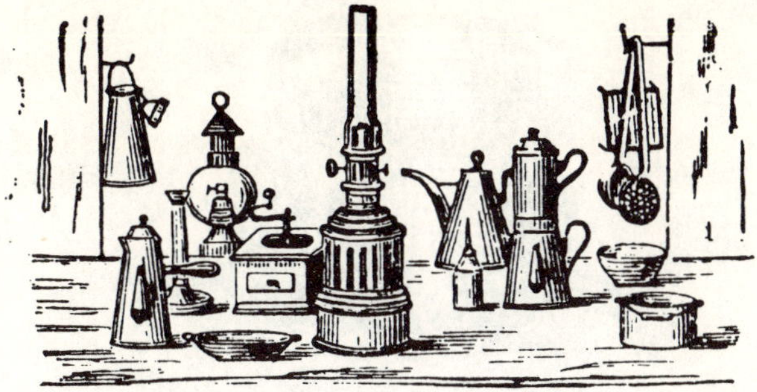

Domestic

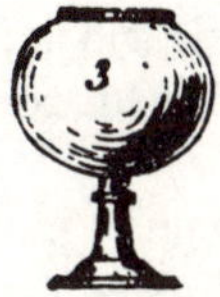

Ink

Take of green vitriol two ounces, of gall-nut three ounces, two ounces of gum Arabic, one ounce of sugar & a half an ounce of blue vitriol; put the whole into a glazed earthenware pot, pour over it a pint of boiling water, set it on hot cinders for twenty-four hours, stirring it from time to time. Let it settle to clarify and boil up the dregs in a pint or so of water for a full half-hour, adding this to the first liquid.

—*Economie Rustique* ou *Notions Simples et Faciles*

To Sweeten Musty Casks

Let the Cask be well Cleaned, then to one that will hold 12 Gall: put in half a pound of Rock Allum, broke; pour on it a Gallon of Boiling Water, stop it close and shake it well and let it remain till Cold, then clean it out and it's fitt for immediate use.

Excellent to Destroy Buggs

½ a pint of the best spirits of Wine, ½ a pint of Spirits of Turpentine, ½ Oz Camphire broke in small pieces, shake it well in a close stopped bottle, use it with a brush or spunge, pour it into the Crevises, shake the bottle.

To recover the Ink of faded Writings

Fill up one quarter of a pint bottle with pounded gall nuts, add spirits of wine or Gin to fill the bottle. Put the letters in a plate & cover it with the mixture; after a short time the writing will become visible.

— *Commonplace Book, circa* 1750

Spirits of wine & sealing wax makes good Varnish.

Receipt for destroying Rats
Take three pennyworth of Oxbane soften it in Water in the Hoven & cut it small then put it in as much water as a Quart of Wheat will soke up depositing the same in the Hoven & to remain untill it is nearly done mixing the same up with a Quarter sugar.

— *Commonplace Book, circa* 1770

To kill Flies take 1 pint of milk ¼ pound raw sugar 2 oz Black pepper boil them 10 min pour it on broad shallow Dishes.

—*Jane Foley's Commonplace Book*

To scour boards
Mix in a saucer three parts of fine sand and one part of lime; dip the scrubbing brush into this and use instead of soap. This will remove grease and whiten the boards, while at the same time it will destroy all insects.

To remove bad smells
Place a jar of permanganate of potash in the vicinity of the obnoxious smell.

To destroy flies

Beer or Treacle in a saucer or treacle smeared on sheets of paper will attract and kill flies. If a small quantity, say the equivalent of a teaspoonful, of carbolic acid be poured on a hot shovel it will drive the flies from the room.

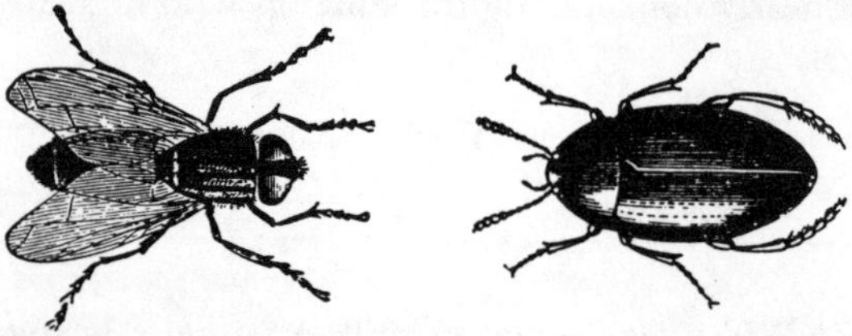

To destroy crickets and beetles

Place a fairly deep saucer of stale beer upon the hearth at night time, and rest three or four sticks upon the edge of the saucer for the insects to crawl up.

To remove scorch marks from linen

Boil ½ pint of vinegar, 2 ozs of fuller's-earth, 1 oz of dried fowl's dung, ½ an oz of soap and the juice of 2 large onions together to the consistency of paste; spread the composition thickly over the damaged part, and if the threads be not actually consumed, after it has been allowed to dry on, and the place has subsequently been washed once or twice, every trace of scorching will disappear.

— *Mrs Beeton*

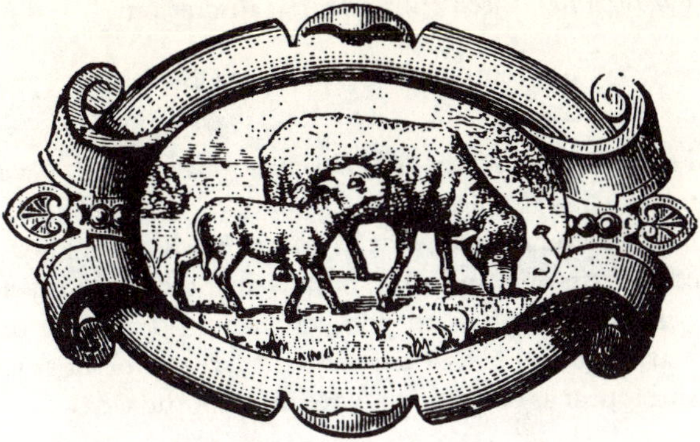

Veterinary

Horse

For a horse that is *prickd in the foot*, clean it out and power in Spts of Turpentine and set them on fire, to crisp the hole And then stuf it up with Lards and salve made of Tar, Turpitine, Lard, Verdegrease, Rosin.

For *Speck in a Horse Eye*, Squart Vinegar into it.

To make a Striking Wild Horse Quiet, Give him about 3 penneyworth of Opium at twise every other Day which will sleep him.

Two ounce of Spts: of Turpentine for a Horse that has the *Belley Ack*.

For the Piles. Pitch Pills taken at discretion.

— *Commonplace Book, circa* 1770

For a Cow or Mare Which having taken a Bad Cold refuseth also its food:
Mix one ounce each of Grains of Paradise, Diaphoretic Antimony and Bay berries in powder, with 2 ounces of Gentian in powder. Stir into a quart of warm ale, with half a pound of Treacle or honey, and repeat as occasion may require, for three days.

To Strengthen and Comfort a Cow after Calving
Give her a loaf of fresh bread, soaked in a liter of good red wine.

For Freckles
Take a wineglass of urine and mix it with a tablespoon of good vinegar. Add a pinch of salt. Let it sit for 24 hours. Then pat it on the freckled skin and leave it for one half hour, and rinse off with plain cold water.

To make ye horse dung water, for Agues and feavers and all distempers.
Take horse dunge and put to it so much Ale as will make it like hasty puding, and put it into your still. Then putt on ye topp one pound of treakell, and a quarter of a pound of genger in powder and the same in sweet anisseeds, and so distill all these together. This water is good for women in labor and in childbed.

A Drench: Take milk and ye Oyl, a good pot. Put Aquavitae to it, and Peper and Brimstone, and Mingle all Together. A pottle at a Time is not too much.

—*A Cordiall Water* M. F. K. Fisher

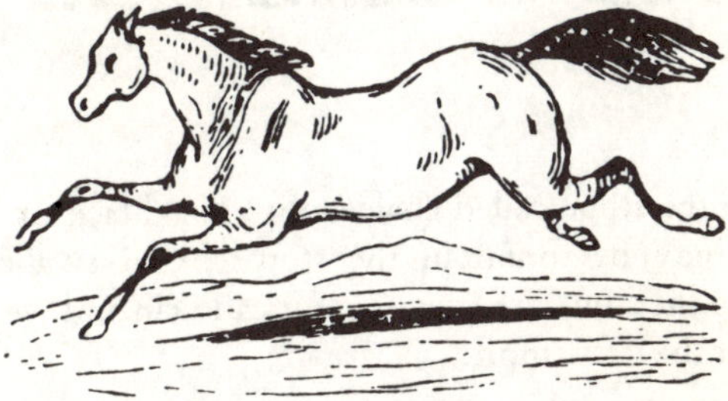

To make a horse do eight times the journey that another could do, without tiring him

Before leaving, mix into his oats a handful of minutely shredded satyrherb; anoint his legs and stomach with venison fat, and mount upon him; bowing low over his left ear, speak softly to him three times, saying the following cabalistic words: *Gaspar, Melchior, Melchisar*. Hang round his neck the fangs of a wolf that has died in the hunt, and leave; your horse will not be in the least tired at the end of the journey.

— *Manualetto dell'Indovino e del Negromante*

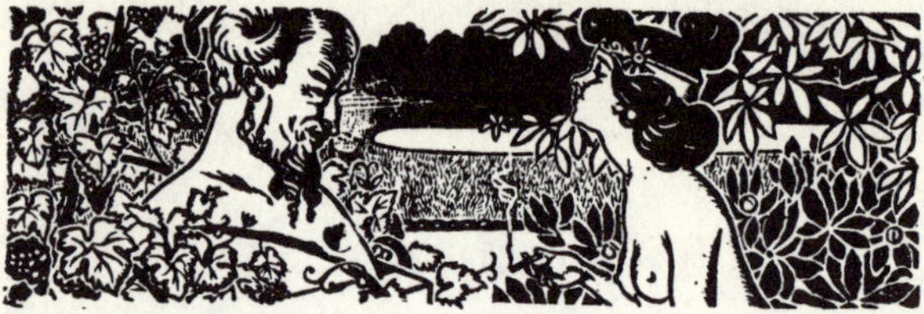

Aphrodisiacs

Take the stone called chalcedony. It is black or red, and may be found in the stomachs of swallows. Wrap the stone in a piece of soft calf skin and wear it under the left armpit.

At sunrise, on a day that promises fine weather, say three times the word TEMON.

Take the marrow of a wolf's foot, mix it with chypre and ambergris and apply it as an unguent to the object of affection.

Take the liver of a sparrow, a pigeon's heart, a hare's kidney, a swallow's womb, and dry and crush them into a powder. Add an equal weight of your own blood. For an infallible potion, dry off the whole and add the resultant powder to a soup.

Take the ash of star-lizard, civet oil and St John's wort oil. Smeared on the toe of the left foot and on the loins, the ointment will serve to reinvigorate. The fat of a young buck, together with civet and ambergris, will do the same.

On the first Friday after a summer's new moon, go out in the middle of the day and find a snake. Cut off its head and bring it away in a fine new silk bag. On arriving home, throw away the stick that you used for killing the snake, throwing it towards the east. Hang up the bag in a dark warm corner. The night after, go in bare feet to a field and before midnight gather up two leaves of white clover, two of red, and six stems of spurge. Bring them back in a new basket. Take a white bud from two rose bushes, a red bud and a young leaf from each, and wrap them in clean parchment. In your own blood, with a fresh goose-quill, write on the parchment the words REVARIN MYRTOL HER KULBATA. Set the basket and the other things at the head of the bed, on a table with a lamp on it that burns for more than three hours.

On rising, spray the leaves and the flowers with cold fresh well water and take them and set them in the corner where the snake's head is drying. Wait until night comes, and then at about eleven o'clock lay out on a table a fresh parchment; by the light of an old church taper held in a silver holder, draw on the parchment a six pointed star.

Get a new chopper, two new knives, a new porcelain bowl, a new clean bottle, a black glass, a flask of cold water, a stick of new wax, a seal, a mortar and a cork.

At midnight, make the sign of the cross three times. Put the snake's head into the mortar with the leaves and flowers and crush them into a paste, heaping them towards the centre of the mortar in a consistent mixture. Put the mortar over the fire until the mixture is dried off, then, while the mortar is still over the flame, pulverise. With the new knives take six drops of your own blood and let them fall into the cup. Add water and then pour the contents of the mortar into the cup, stirring and boiling as you do. Then take three of your hairs, calcine them and throw them into the cup. Do the same with the parchment and the bag. Pour the whole into the bottle, adding water until it overflows.

Cork it and seal it and place it in the bed. Put out the light, pray, and go to sleep.

After three days, kept in the dark, the brew is ready. Taken with drink or food, five drops for men, three for women.

— *Albertus Maximus*

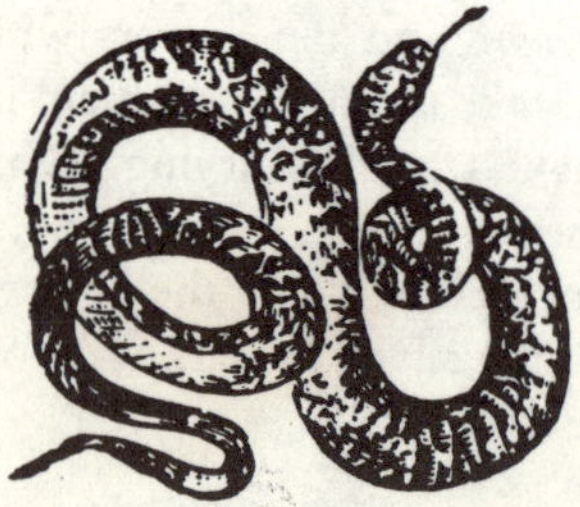

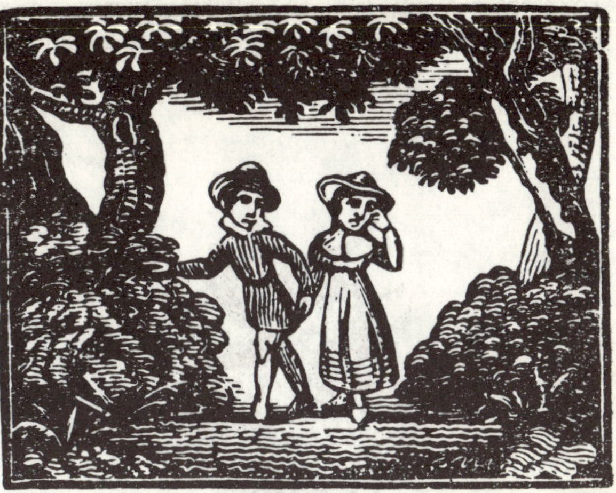

Cut into small pieces the shoots of the vajnasunhi plant, dip them into red arsenic and sulphur mixed, and dry them seven times. Take the powder that is left and burn it, at night. If, when you look at the smoke from it, you can see a golden moon through it, your amatory episode will be successful.

Vigor is increased by a brew consisting of rice with sparrows' eggs, boiled in milk together with honey and ghee.

Take one hundred and fifty seeds of the inner bark of the Moh tree (Bassia Latifolia), heap in a mortar and beat. Drink it in cow's milk.

To prepare a powerful and alluring incense, mix equal quantities of cardamom seeds, oliba, and the plant ghrurwel, sandalwood, flower of jasmine and Bengal madder.

— *Kama Sutra*

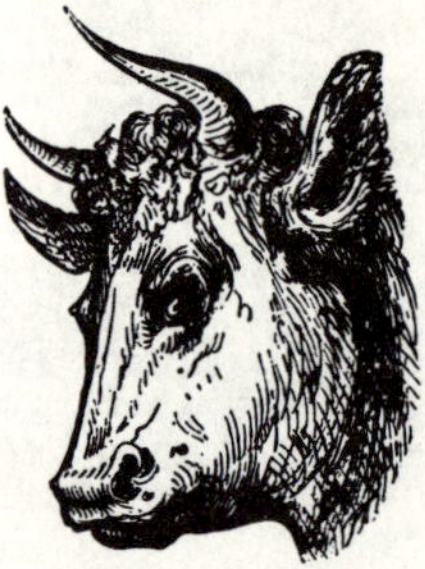

To make a pie of bulls' testicles, take four of them and boil them in water and salt. Cut them in slices, sprinkle them with white pepper, salt, cinnamon and nutmeg. Prepare separately a mince of lambs' kidney, gravy, three slices of lean ham, a good pinch of chopped marjoram, thyme, and three cloves. Prepare the pastry for the pie. Then begin to make a layer on your pie dish with the ham, then a layer of slices of testicles, sprinkle well with the mince, and so on. Before shutting the pie, add a glass of wine. Put it in the oven and serve hot.

— *Cartoleomeo Scappi*
(Private chef to His Holiness Pope Pius V)

Take a large olive, remove the stone and fill it with a paste made of anchovy, capers and oil. Take a trussed and boned garden warbler and put the stuffed olive inside it. Then put the garden warbler inside a fat young wheat-ear. Then take the wheat-ear bird and put it in a boned lark. Put the stuffed lark into a boned thrush, the thrush into a fat quail, the quail to be wrapped in vine leaves and put inside a boned lapwing. Then put the lapwing inside a boned golden plover, the plover into a fat boned red-legged partridge, the partridge into a young boned woodcock. Roll the woodcock in breadcrumbs.

Put the bread-crumbed woodcock into a boned teal and then put the teal into a boned guinea-fowl. Lard the guinea fowl and put it inside a young boned tame duck. Then take the duck and put it into a fat boned fowl. Put the fowl into a well-hung pheasant. Put the pheasant into a fat wild goose, the goose into a turkey, and the turkey into a bustard.

Having thus prepared your roast, put it in a saucepan with onions stuffed with cloves, carrots, small squares of ham, celery and mignonette.

Close off the saucepan with a pastry and set it for ten hours over a gentle fire, making sure that the heat penetrates evenly.

When it is cooked, remove the pastry, remove the grease if there is any, set on a hot dish, and eat.

—*Le Parfait Cuisinier* A. T. Raimbault 1814

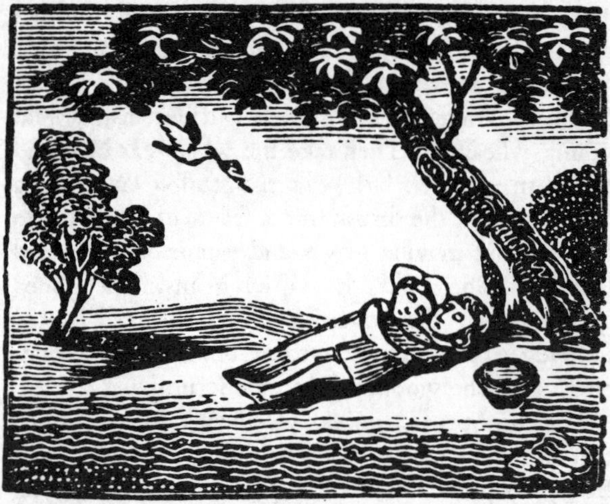

Anaphrodisiacs

If thou wilt that a woman bee not visious nor desire men, take the private members of a Woolfe, and the haires which doe grow on the cheekes or eyebrowes, of him, and the haires which bee under his bearde and burne it all, and give it to her to drinke, when she knoweth not, and she shall desire no other man.

Take the powdered genitalia of a timid bull and make from them a soup, including in it also veal, purslain and lettuce.

— *Albertus Maximus*

Against love.
If you wish to stop loving someone unworthy of your love, take the following potion: on Monday, when the full moon begins to wane, at midnight, when the cock's crowing has banished the demons of the night, leave your house and betake yourself to the banks of a rivulet, to a pond, or to a marsh; arrived there, go barefoot, and pick three flowers, saying each time: *O pheboea senescente! remissio amoris sit inter nos.* Return home before the cock crows and put the three little flowers in a phial with half a spoonful of fine white vinegar. Place the phial for thirteen nights in your window under the influence of the stars. During this time, observe a rigorous fast, abstaining also from any form of fermented liquor, or similar; on the thirteenth day place in the phial three spoonfuls of autumn-gathered honey, adding to it a glassful of the water from the rivulet at whose banks you gathered the flowers. At the end of your fast, at midday, drink the potion, reciting the while the above-mentioned magic words. You will instantly turn against the person, and without looking at them – and above all without touching them – go in anger with them and cease to love them.
This potion has the additional virtue of curing obesity and preventing attacks of apoplexy.

— *Manualetto dell'Indovino e del Negromante*

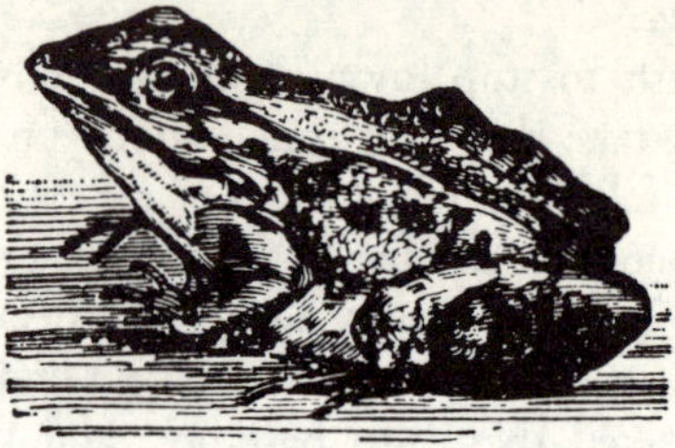

Potions

(It must here be pointed out that persons of wisdom and prudence do well to abstain from the making of potions, whether for themselves or for others. This proceeds (1) from the fact that occasional grave results may follow from the taking of these beverages, which, in such cases, may amount to poisonings, which the law punishes with justice and severity. We refer to certain potions whose constituents have been described in a number of ignorant and imprudent publications, whereas with those to be found here we have taken care scrupulously to avoid all poisonous substances such as, for example, tincture of cantharides and of apples, cream of mushrooms, metallic oxides, etc.; (2) that it is known that Night Spirits sometimes strangle those individuals who seek to involve themselves in the making of potions without being truly accepted members of the High Chapter of wizards and spellmakers – a matter of very common occurence.)

Against a woman's infidelity. Take of the hide of a wolf the hair that surrounds the eyes, that which encircles his throat, and his whiskers, and reduce to ashes by means of calcination; mix a pinch of this in a glass of wine without her knowledge and have her drink it; she will not attempt to cuckold her husband again.

Against the infidelity of husbands. The dorsal marrow of a wolf, calcinated and used in similar manner, renders men faithful to their wives.

— *Manualetto dell'Indovino e del Negromante*

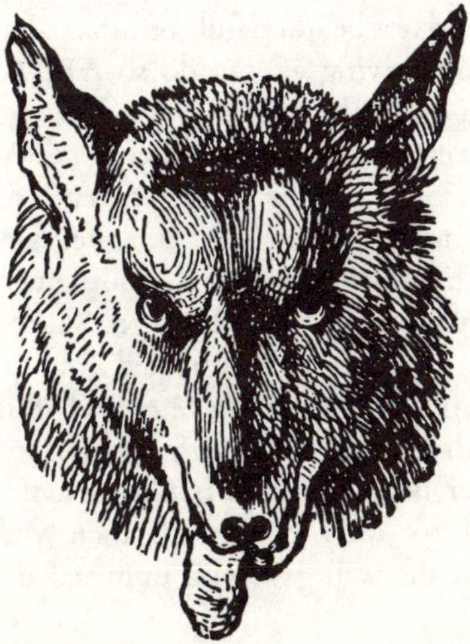

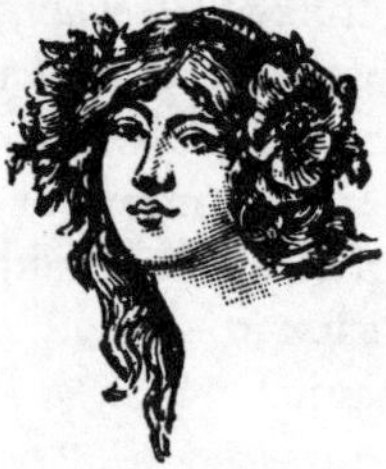

To gain the favours of a lady. Take an ounce and a half of candied sugar. With a pestle and mortar that has never been used before, grind it into a coarse powder. Do this on a Wednesday morning, saying while you are grinding ABRASAX, ABRACADABRA. Turn out the sugar into a litre of good white wine and place the wine in a cellar or in a dark cupboard for twenty-seven days. Each morning, take the bottle, which should not be quite full, and shake it vigorously for a minute, saying as you do so ABRASAX. Do the same again in the evening, but shaking the bottle for three minutes, and saying three times ABRACADABRA. Finally, on the twenty-seventh day, decant the potion into a bottle of Champagne. As you do so, add, three times, three grains of white mustard – and the potion is ready. On the next Sunday, on one pretext or another invite the lady in question to lunch at your house, tête-à-tête, and if she comes, have her drink as much of the potion as she likes, making her believe that it is Champagne. She will need to drink only half of it, then you may be certain that she will give you unmistakable signs of her love.

To cure somebody of drunkenness. Take the blood of an eel. Drip three drops into a bottle of wine, saying in a loud voice ASTAROT; then two more drops, saying ASSAIBI, and lastly another three saying BACNOE. Then form in the air the cabalistic numbers 3, 5, 7; have the drunkard drink this wine, and he will not get drunk for more than a month.

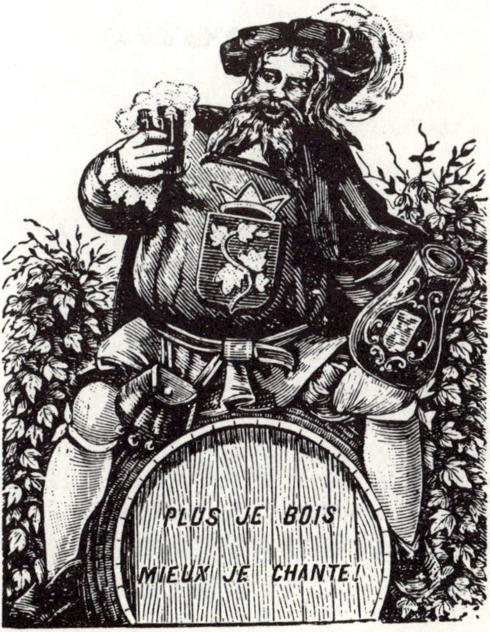

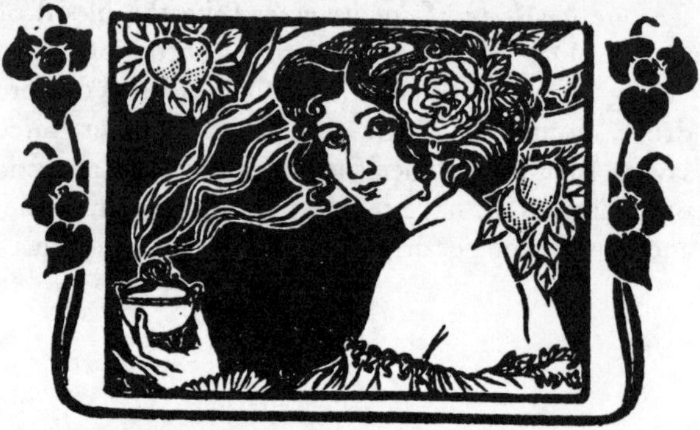

Cosmetic

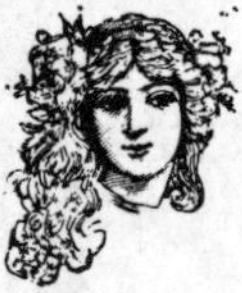

To make the Hair grow thick
Take Rosemary, Maidenhair, Southernwood, Myrtle-berries, Hazelbark, of each two ounces, burn these to ashes on a clean hearth, or in an oven, put these ashes in white Wine, and wash the hair daily at the root, and keep it cut pretty short.

— *Commonplace Book of Elizabeth Plowman*

Anti-freckle lotion

Mix 2 ozs of tincture of benzoin, 1 oz of tincture of tolu; ½ a drachm of oil of rosemary well in a corked bottle. When required for use, add a teaspoonful of the mixture to a wineglassful of water, and apply the lotion where required night and morning, gently dabbing it in with a soft linen.

To make cold cream

A very simple way of making this is to put 1 lb. of lard in a basin and fill up with boiling water. When cold, and the lard has risen to the top, take it off and repeat the process. When cold again, whisk it up with a paper knife until it becomes a perfectly smooth cream, then add enough essence of lemon to give it perfume.

Areca nut tooth-powder

Reduce to a very fine charcoal 2½ ozs of areca nut, and pound as finely as possible another ½ oz in its raw state, then mix with 1 oz of finely powdered cuttlefish bone, and flavour with cloves or cassia according to taste.

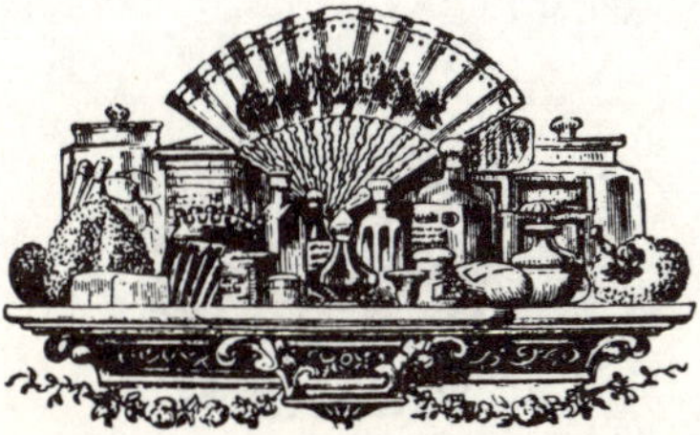

Attar of Roses

(Two hundred thousand well-grown roses are required to produce half an ounce of attar; and this quantity, when manufactured, sells, if genuine, for about £12 at the English warehouses. It is very difficult, however, to obtain the genuine article, as even the original manufacturers adulterate it.)

Fill a large earthen jar, or other vessel, with the leaves of rose-flowers picked over and freed from all dust and dirt. Pour upon them as much pure spring water as will cover them, and from sunrise to sunset, for 6 or 7 days in succession, set the vessel where it will receive the sun's rays. At the end of the fourth day a number of particles of a fine yellow oily matter will float on the surface, which, after a day or two, will gather into a scum. This is the attar of roses. It must be taken up as often as it appears, with a piece of cotton wool tied to a stick, and squeezed from this into a small phial, which must be kept corked and tied over.

— *Mrs Beeton*

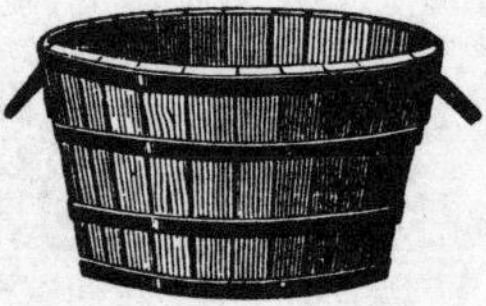

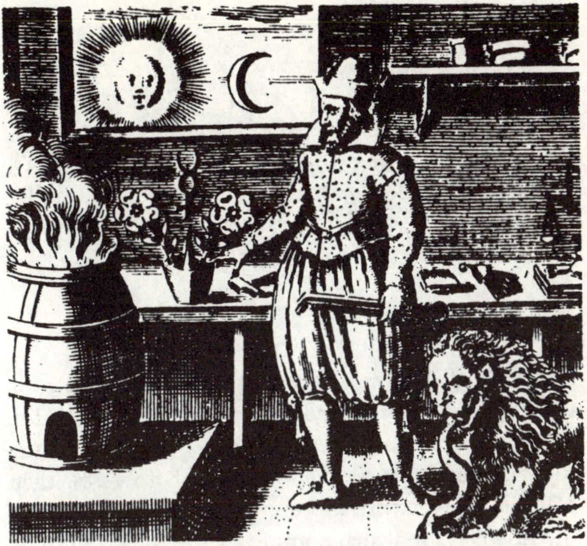

Miscellaneous

To Cure Blight in Trees

1 lb Flour of Sulphur; 1 Gallon Urine. Mix these well together, add as much Cow dung as will make it the consistence of Paint in January after you have cut your Trees before the bud begins to swell paint the whole tree thoroughly this will prevent Mildew. Fumagate the Tree with Tobacco washing it well the next day with Lime Water with infusion of Tobacco.

— *Commonplace Book, circa* 1750

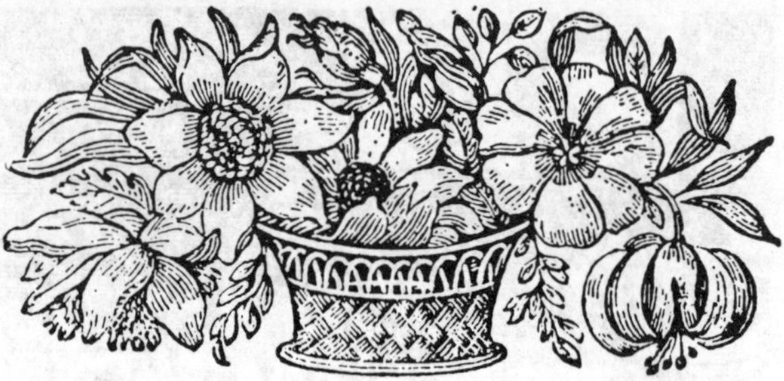

A Sallat of floweres: Take of floweres, primrose, cowslip and clove-gillyfloweres, a deep basketful. Cut off their stalkes. Prepare a large pot, strew a little sugar in the bottom, then a layer of floweres, then cover that layer with more sugar, then lay another of the floweres, and then another of the sugar, and this do above one another until the pot be filled to the verie top.

Then press the floweres and sugar hard down with your hand. Then take a sharpe and bitter wine and pour into the pot until it floats above the top layer. Then set in a dry temperature and seal the pot well. Then eat the salat at your pleasure, for it will last fresh until the floweres come again.

– 17th Century recipe quoted in *Herbal Handbook for Everyone*
Juliette de Baïracli Levy
(Faber and Faber)

The Traveller's Staff

On the eve of All Saints, cut a rod of elder to make a staff. Remove the pith from the inside of the rod and fit the lower end of the rod with a metal ferrule. Then take the two eyes of a wolf, the tongue and heart of a dog, three lizards, three nightingales' hearts, and dry them thoroughly in the sun, sprinkling them with finely powdered saltpetre. Put them into the hollow of the rod, finishing off with seven leaves of verbena and a multicoloured stone from the nest of an owl. Seal off the end with a plug of clay or other material. This staff will save you, during your journey, from every kind of danger and inconvenience, and will protect you from robbers, from assassins, from wild beasts, from mad dogs, from vipers, etc.

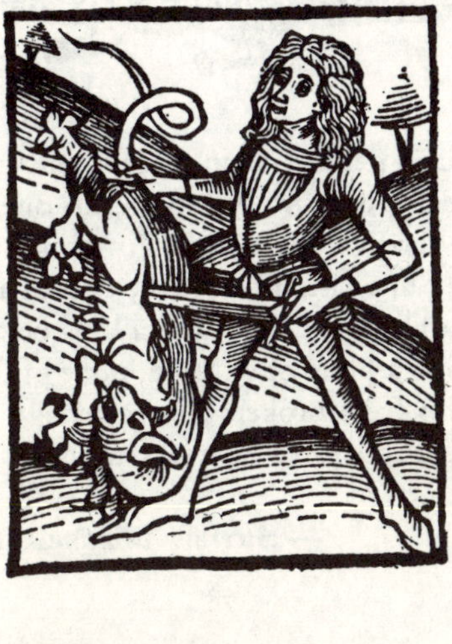

To stop frogs croaking
There are old castles surrounded by moats and houses situated in the neighbourhood of marshes or surrounded by water where the racket set up by frogs makes it impossible to drop off to sleep. Only the Lamp of Alberto can put a stop to it. This is the way to prepare it: melt together some sun-blanched wax with crocodile fat – but as crocodile fat is not easy to come by in this country whale oil may be used as a substitute; into the mixture place a thickish wick; light the lamp and place it on the bank of the water: the frogs will immediately stop croaking.

— *Manualetto dell'Indovino e del Negromante*

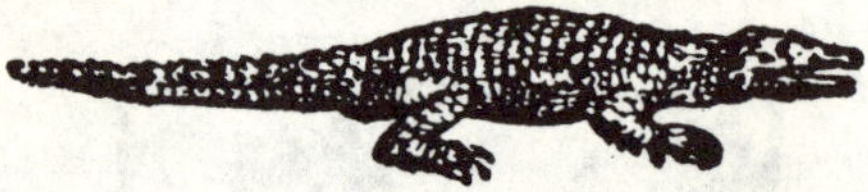

If one gathers heliotrope in August and wraps it up in a bay-leaf with a wolf's tooth, no-one can speak an angry word to the wearer. Put under the pillow it will bring in a vision before the eyes of a man who has been robbed, the thief and all his belongings. If it be set up in a place of worship, none of the women present who have broken their marriage vows will be able to quit the place till it be removed.

—*Albertus Maximus* (1193-1280)

There are some perfumes or suffumagations, which make men speak in their sleep, walk and do those things that are done by men that are awake and often, what when awake they cannot do or dare do. Others again make men hear horrid sounds, or delightful sounds, noises, and the like.

A perfume made of hempseeds, of the seeds of fleawort, violett roots and parsley maketh men to see things to come and is available for prophesie. A marvellous efficacious fumigation to cause a man to see visions in the air and elsewhere: take coriander, and henbane and the skin that is within the pound-garnet (pomegranate) and the fumigation is finished as you desire.

To see future events: fumigate yourself with linseed and seed of psellium or with violet roots and wild parsley.

From two sixteenth century writers

The commonplace books from which extracts are reproduced are items from private collections. The publishers acknowledge the kind co-operation of Mrs Kathleen Brown of Uckfield, and Mrs Alice Buckley of West Hoathly in making them available for transcription. Translations from *Economie Rustique* and from *Manualetto dell' Indovino* are copyright by Maurice Rickards, who also devised the cover design.